The G-Spot, The Clitoris & A Woman's Orgasm

The Secret Connection Between All Three

by T.K. Hereford

Preliminaries

I know how eager you are to get right to the heart of this subject. I promise you, we will get there in due course. However, before we get to that part, there are a few preliminaries that we need to discuss. These form the foundations of our discussion.

Definition of an "Erogenous Zone"

We are going to begin this journey together by defining an "erogenous zone". It will help shortly.

To understand a word, it is often useful to look at how it came to be. In English, so many of our words have roots in either Greek or Latin. "Erogenous" is no different. This is a combination of two Greek words. These are "eros" and "genes". Eros is the Greek word for love that implies intimacy, romance and erotic desire. In fact, "erotic", in the English language also draws root from "eros" and should give you clearer idea of the type of love I mean. "Genes" means "born of" or "producing" in English. As such, one could read "erogenous" as "love producing" if one were so inclined.

This agrees with the commonly accepted English definition. That definition, to paraphrase, is an area of the body, which, upon stimulation can result in sexual arousal. Note that I did not say "causes an orgasm". That's not part of the definition. An erogenous zone is nothing more than a part of the body that can be stimulated to produce sexual arousal.

Commonly accepted body parts that fall within this definition are nipples, toes, lips, the clitoris, the penis, testicles, breasts, buttocks, earlobes, thighs, both sets of vaginal lips, the back of the neck, armpits and the anus. That is by no means an exhaustive list. I'm just listing a few.

Just to make sure that we're clear, I'll repeat myself. An erogenous zone, in it's commonly accepted usage, is nothing more than a part of the body that, when stimulated, can result in sexual arousal. As we move forward, please keep this definition in mind.

Defining The G-Spot

Before I can move on to convincing you that the G-Spot doesn't exist, I need to describe what it's supposed to be. Many of you will have preconceptions and for a lot of you this may be redundant, but I want to, again, make sure we are all on the same page so ideas flow logically.

The G-Spot, as originally described, is supposed to be an

erogenous zone located on the front wall of a woman's vaginal canal. It's described as being a few inches inside and along the line of her urethra. A picture is worth a thousand words and it is no less true in this case. In the image below, the purported location of the G-Spot is marked by the black arrow in the diagram, along the front wall of the vagina along the line of the urethra. Please note it's location.

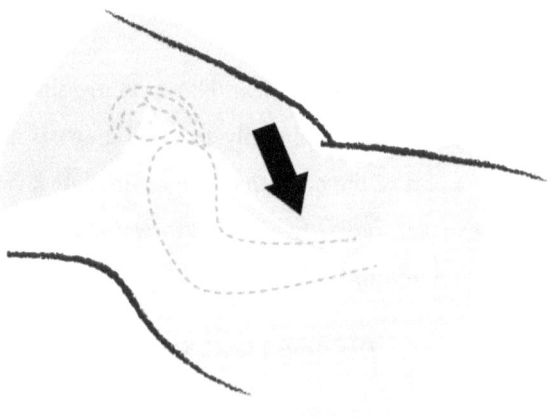

As we move forward, this will be our definition of G-Spot. Again, that is an erogenous zone located on the front wall of a woman's vaginal canal along the line of her urethra.

Where Did The G-Spot Theory Come From?

There are two men, mind you men, who bear responsibility for what we can call the G-Spot today. The first of these was Dr. Sigmund Freud and the other was Dr. Ernst Grafenburg. Incidentally, it's the "G" in Grafenburg that gives the G-Spot it's name.

Freud was the first of these two men to write and as such, I will start off with him. Writing at the tail end of the Victorian era in 1905, Freud was really one of the first researchers to begin to attempt to reason his way through the labyrinth that is human sexuality. Many of his conclusions at this point have been dismissed by current researchers. Among these was his research into a common condition of the time known as frigidity. Frigidity was the commonly held belief that if a woman could not orgasm as a result of intercourse, there was something wrong with her.

Freud addressed frigidity in his "Three Essays On The Theory Of Sexuality". In my opinion, anyone wishing to truly understand the roots of the G-Spot phenomenon should read this work outright. This work is one of the foundations of the belief that women could and should, as part of the natural developmental process, be able to orgasm vaginally, through sexual intercourse. (For the record, I completely disagree with this and I'll tell you why shortly.) Unfortunately, it was just plain wrong, but it sent out a clarion message to women around the world that if you couldn't orgasm as a result of sexual intercourse, you were broken. After all, Freud was a doctor and doctors are presumed to know where of they speak.

Unfortunately, in my opinion, Freud was off the mark. Freud did agree that young, prepubescent girls can and did give themselves orgasms by stimulating their clitorises. However, he argued that as part of the maturing process, a woman's sexual center should transfer from her clitoris to her vagina. He reasoned that since the vagina, and not the clitoris is the part of a woman's anatomy most involved in the process of sexual reproduction, it should naturally take center stage. As it's the most important part of a woman's genitals as well, he reasoned, it should be from here, like the penis in men, that a sexually mature woman derives her pleasure.

I want to pause here for a minute to draw special attention to one of the things Freud said. That is, the fact that a woman, upon maturing should move her pleasure center from her clitoris to her vagina. Even for the Victorian era with its myriad of...questionable beliefs, this borders on the absurd, in my opinion. Freud, a doctor, threw this idea out there, said that a woman who do it was somehow defective, yet offered no insight into how this process was supposed to happen. Additionally, he cited no evidence that led him to this conclusion nor any studies that supported the idea. No one ever told me how I was supposed to switch my sexual focus from my clit to my vagina. It didn't happen on it's own to my knowledge, but I have to assume that's normal, since I never met a woman that it has happened to. How curious.

Now, I do have to concede that Freud was writing during a period of hidden sexuality. The Victorian period was well known for sexual repression and forced social modesty. It was hard for me to get friends of mine to discuss their orgasm habits and G-Spot beliefs in an open manner in the present day. Prior to 1905 when he wrote, I would imagine that it was downright impossible for Dr. Freud to get women to talk to him openly and honestly about their orgasm habits, let alone to let him go poking around down there to do a little empirical research to back up his ideas. If he had, I wonder if his conclusions would have stayed the same.

That being said, the idea that a woman can somehow, magically move the major pleasure producing parts of her anatomy from one spot to another seems to be an odd assertion. Human development takes place on its own without any input, as a general rule, from a body's owner. Men's testicles drop with no thought of theirs to encourage them, just the same as women grow breasts and get their first period. If it's supposed to happen in human development, it just sort of happens. The failure for this "movement" to occur in the vast majority of women was not taken up by Freud. The idea that women can and should orgasm during sex through only the stimulation of their vaginas was taken up, however, and made popular, along with the idea that any woman who could not was somehow defective.

Freud didn't suggest how or by what organ women should be able to orgasm vaginally, he just said that they should. Where he left off, another doctor, Dr. Ernst Grafenburg picked up several decades later.

Dr. Grafenburg, a urologist, described an erogenous zone that he believed he'd found in 1950. His work, "The Role Of The Urethra In Female Orgasm" (another one everyone should read) described an erogenous zone along the anterior wall of a woman's vagina along the line of her urethra. Grafenburg believed that the urethra played an important role in female orgasm, like it does in men. The urethra, is after all, how sperm is delivered from the male reproductive system to the female.

In his article, to paraphrase, Grafenburg said that the orgasms that were produced from stimulating this particular erogenous zone did not result in muscle contraction like those that occur during an orgasm produced from clitoral stimulation. In my opinion, that is a bit of a problem. Any woman who has ever had an orgasm, and any man for that fact, will attest that there are powerful muscular contractions that go along with them. In fact, in most cases, the clinical definition of an orgasm includes muscle contractions as a given. Where were these in Grafenburg's experiments?

If the women in his studies were indeed having very real orgasms, why then were there no muscular contractions?

It doesn't matter. Like with Freud, the world picked up on Grafenburg's research, coupled it with Freud's assertion that women should be able to orgasm vaginally and ran with it. You as a woman, the world loves to tell women, should be able to cum through your vagina, by using your G-spot and if you can't there is something wrong with you.

These men, in my opinion, were both half right. I believe, like Freud said, that a woman can orgasm during sexual intercourse. I have personal experience enough to believe this to be true. However, I disagree with his belief that it's a natural part of a woman's sexuality and should happen automatically with sexual maturity. Grafenburg, on the other hand, I think was on to something when he talked about women in his study responding pleasurably to stimulation along the front wall of the vagina. However, I don't think what he found was any new erogenous zone, or mysterious spot.

Anatomy Textbooks Do Not Show The G-Spot

In my early research I found something startling that I feel needed to be put very early in this book.

If you go and walk into a college library, even one for medical students, and you go and browse through the textbooks you will not find the G-Spot on the illustrations. Everything else is there. The vagina, the labia minora, majora, ovaries, uterus, fallopian tubes, etc, etc, etc. Everything that you would expect to find in an anatomy textbook is listed. However, the G-Spot isn't. It's simply not there.

Why?

It's not there, because to medical science, the G-Spot remains as elusive as the Loch Ness monster. There's no structure that's consistent in the human form to identify. Everyone has a heart. It can be found. Everyone has a liver. It's there. It can be identified, measured and evaluated. If you're a woman you have a clitoris and a vagina. Every man has a penis. The same can be said for all the other identifiable parts of the human body. They can be identified, measured, quantified and as a result, are in the hallowed volumes of anatomy that are used to educate medical professionals.

The G-Spot enjoys no such distinction. If you were to dissect a human cadaver in a medical anatomy class, you would never be able to find the G-Spot, even though you now know exactly where to look. There's no special tissue, no organ, nothing consistently distinguishable at all at that location.

Gynecologists are just as unlikely to point out the G-Spot out for you. Remember, they're doctors too. They were educated by those medical books that omit the G-Spot.

As far as medical science is concerned, the G-Spot is an unconfirmed story at best. It's a subject to explore, but it has eluded doctors to this day.

For me, this was one of the most damning bits of information concerning my belief in the G-Spot. If medical science could not point to it, isolate it, photograph it or conclusively demonstrate its existence, something, in my opinion, was wrong. Medical science can do wonderful, wonderful things. It can manipulate brain chemicals, clone sheep, create synthetic blood cells, perform laproscopic surgery on the heart and other organs, and more other miracles than I can list. Don't even get me started on MRIs and CAT scans. Using these technologies, pathologists can tell how a five thousand year old mummy died.

How then, with all the space aged, advanced technology that medical science can bring to bear, can this seemingly easy to find little pleasure button escape detection?

For me, in my own head, the answer had to be that there was nothing there to find. If medicine couldn't find it, I reasoned, there had to be something fundamentally wrong with the theory as a whole. After I learned this, any remaining belief I had in the G-Spot just crumbled.

The Fact Remained That Women Can Cum Vaginally

In all the science classes I ever took, I recall being told that scientific inquiry began with observation. We see something happening and then we attempt to explain it. In the inquiry that I was conducting, the observed reality was that women, at times, myself included, could be stimulated to orgasm during sex. There was just too much personal experience and candid evidence to dismiss it all out of hand.

In those same science classes, I also recall that when trying to explain an observed occurrence, we put forward theories. The most popular theory, explaining this observation, in my opinion, today, is the G-Spot. The thought goes that there's some magically sensitive little bundle of nerves somewhere in a woman's vagina that a man only needs to rub against to give her orgasms.

I've never found my G-Spot. I have never met anyone who has told me that they have found their G-Spot. Men, are excluded for the simple fact that bravado and confusion make their testimony unreliable. I've never met a woman who has told me that they have found their G-Spot. Although, I have found women who had been able to orgasm during sex. Additionally, medicine failed to show me clearly where the G-Spot was as well. All off this added up to a lot of doubt in my head that the G-Spot was anything real.

But , there was a problem. The fact remained that women

can and do orgasm during sex.

When one theory explaining the observation fails, as the G-Spot theory had in my own head, we have to offer another theory. A long time back, people believed the sun rotated around the Earth. It was a great theory, it just didn't work. People would make predictions along that line of thinking that didn't come true. Those failings exposed the flaws of the theory. Eventually, the theory was thrown out and replaced with one that could accurately explain and predict celestial observations and events.

That's what I did too. I threw out my belief in the G-Spot as an explanation of how women can cum during sex. There were just too many holes and inconsistencies for me. Enough was enough. There had to be something else that made sense. There had to be something that I could test out in my bedroom with my partner, that I could replicate time and time again, that made sense of facts and observations.

That's what I think I found.

I think I found an explanation of how I could orgasm during sex, without relying on the G-Spot theory, that made sense logically, and that my partner and I could replicate in the bedroom. There wasn't a trick. There wasn't a gimmick. There were just a few crucial bits of information that got left out of my sex ed classes.

The rest of this book, will be dedicated to that information and applying it in your own life.

The Clitoris & The Simple Truth

I've already mentioned how Freud argued that for a woman to mature, sexually speaking, she needed to transfer the "locus" of her sexuality away from her clitoris, to her vagina. He reasoned, that since the vagina plays the most important part in sexual reproduction, in a woman's anatomy, that this should also be the well spring of her pleasure as well.

For me, there was only one problem with this thinking. Freud assumed that pleasure and function go hand in hand in a woman's body as much as they do in a man's. I believe they don't.

What do I mean by this?

A man's job, biologically speaking, in sexual reproduction is to provide sperm to a woman. That's it. He accomplishes this through orgasm, which is pleasurable. From an evolutionary standpoint, this make total sense. Things that feel good encourage us to do it more. Orgasms would seem to be pleasurable to encourage full release of sperm to a woman during sex. While there is sperm present in the pre-orgasm secretions of a man, it's much, much less likely that he will impregnate his partner without full release. Basically, he can't do the job unless he orgasms and the pleasure is there to encourage him to do just that. It's worked for as long as humans have walked the Earth.

That is not the case at all with a woman.

Women can indeed become pregnant and give birth to healthy, beautiful children without an orgasm ever entering into the picture. Put in short, an orgasm is completely unnecessary to a woman's biological role in sexual reproduction.

At first, when I was reasoning all this out, I was tempted to make the assumption that the clitoris had developed along the same "pleasure to perform a task" lines as the penis. That is to say, the pleasure encouraged women to have sex more, and as a result, more reproduction occurred. But I was forced to face facts.

The clitoris's role in sexual reproduction is tangential at best. Clitoral stimulation during intercourse just doesn't happen easily enough or routinely to seem connected. If the clitoris's purpose was to produce physical pleasure during sex, to encourage more sex, it honestly seemed to be doing a really bad job of it.

On the one hand, if every woman's clitoris was located in her vagina and orgasm during sex was in the 80-90% range, the argument for the pleasure encouraging procreation argument could be made. But that's not where the clitoris is. It's outside the vagina, only adjacent to it and is all too often completely unstimulated during sex. Plus the orgasm during sex rate is nowhere near 80% of the time as I'm sure any woman reading this will agree.

I also did a little thinking about the deplorable practice of removing the clitoris that is a common cultural practice in many parts of Saharan and Northern Africa. This is often done with the aim of removing sexual pleasure and consequently sexual temptation and is sadly looked upon as a routine occurrence in many young woman's life.

As repugnant as I personally find this practice to be, the tradition did offer me some further insight in my thinking. My examination of this practice actually convinced me of the separation between pleasure and reproduction where the clitoris is concerned.

The practice of removing the clitoris is a long standing and deeply rooted one in many areas of Sub-Saharan Africa. There are records of the British attempting to stop the practice during the colonial period of Africa as well. I personally believe the practice should be outlawed and abandoned and I support efforts to outlaw it in the United States, Europe, Canada and Australia. That being said, the practice did show that the cultural practice of removing the clitoris did not cause the extinction of the culture that practiced it. On the contrary, many of Northern and Saharan African countries where this practice is still prevalent, have some of the highest birth rates in the world according to the Organization of Economic Cooperation and Development.

This was a big eye opener for me when I reasoned it all out. Men, need to orgasm to do their job in continuing the species. As such, it should come naturally during sex. Surprise! It does. Men never seem to need to figure anything out. There's not trick to it. Half the time, I'll bet men don't even get their pants all the way off before they cum in a woman for the first time. They stick it in the first time, pump a little and bam, they're done. But it felt great. They want to do it again. They didn't need anyone to teach them. They didn't need a book, a magazine, a diagram or a chart. They just did it. It just came naturally.

Women need a lot more help, it would seem to figure out how to cum during sex. That seemed odd. Mother Nature is really good at making necessary things simple. We don't even think about breathing. Your heart just beats and beats and beats. A woman gets her first period, just because it's time. No one asked her. Things that should happen, from a purely biological necessity standpoint, just happen. Then, there's a woman's orgasm. During masturbation there's no real trick to it. We all focus on our clits and that's that. But as far a sex is concerned, we need diagrams and someone to let us in on "the secret". I'm sure you know what I mean. You bought this book for that very reason.

So I sat down and I did a little thinking as to why this might be the case. My thinking seemed to create a logical conundrum. If a woman was "supposed" to cum during sex, it should be easier. This didn't add up and needed to be reconciled. Here's what I came up with and it worked for me and sent me off in, what I believe, was the right direction.

Let's talk about nipples for a minute.

Men have nipples. It's a fact. But they do nothing. The just lay there. They're perfectly functionless. Sometimes they're fun to pierce and I admit men would look weird without them, but they don't do anything. Nothing at all. In women, of course they are extremely functional. No baby could eat if women didn't have functional nipples. But men don't need them at all, at any point in their lives.

Why then, are they there?

Men have nipples as a result of their origin as a blank human embryo. All babies, whether male of female, start developing the same way, to a point and then gender specific attributes begin to develop. But up to a point, we exist as a "blank" human embryo with neither physical characteristics. The tissue that forms either the clitoris or the penis is there before the sex characteristics develop and so are the nipples.

Mother Nature seemed so concerned with making sure that female humans wound up with nipples, so they could nurse their babies, that she went ahead and programmed that part of our DNA on a very, very basic level. She was so afraid that it was going to get left out that she made it one of the first things to form. She didn't even seem to care if the finished human would need them. Yes, as a result, men wound up with useless nipples that do nothing but grow those mysteriously long, curly hairs. But, in doing so, Mother Nature made sure every human who needed nipples to get some actual work done had some.

The clitoris, and a woman's ability to orgasm, I believe fall into a similar category. They are there, because men need the clitoris to form into a sperm delivering penis so they can fulfill their "biologic role" in sexual reproduction. Like nipples, Mother Nature seemed to want to make sure anyone who needed these parts and abilities to get the job done, had them, regardless of whether or not she had to hand out a few extras.

All of this thinking and reasoning, allowed me to cut the Gordian knot that led Freud, to what I believe, were off conclusions. A woman's pleasure center doesn't migrate to her vagina upon reaching sexual maturity, because in women, pleasure and function aren't supposed to naturally go together.

Instead of trying to reconcile why they don't go together, I found it easier and much more logical to just assume that they don't. That is to say, that a woman's orgasm is not necessary, or intended by design to happen.

Now just because it's not technically necessary, doesn't make it useless, pointless or something to ignore. I know plenty of men who draw a lot of pleasure from nipple play. It's great foreplay and a lot of fun. An orgasm in women does much the same in men. It feels great. It bonds us to our partners. It creates feelings of closeness, intimacy and connection. Endorphins are released. Mental health is improved. Calmness prevails. Small wonder that women love cumming just as much as men do. But, that still doesn't mean that it's necessary- from a technical point of view.

When I sat down in a bean bag chair and reasoned all this out, I had a bit of an epiphany, that pointed me in the right direction, like I've said. If the orgasm function is only necessary for men, and men orgasm via their penises, then the orgasm function in women, all of it, should be contained in a woman's analogous organ to the penis. That is to say - the clitoris. There's no second orgasm function in men and building one in women, especially when the orgasm function itself seems unnecessary to a woman's role in sexual reproduction made no sense.

Logically speaking, at that point, I began to suspect that the clitoris had a few secrets that I needed to unravel. As I am apt to do, I hit the books and did some more research. What I found certainly got left out of my sex education. The clitoris is not a popular subject with gym and health teachers, but there is a lot more to it than I had ever been led to believe.

The Wonderful, Truly Misunderstood Clitoris

The clitoris is much more than most people think. Like an iceberg, most of what the clitoris is actually lies below the surface. Additionally, I believe, there is much, much more sensitivity and ability to offer orgasms than most people realize. I'm not going to keep you waiting. I'm going to put my A+ material right up front. Let's look at the clitoris.

Here it is!

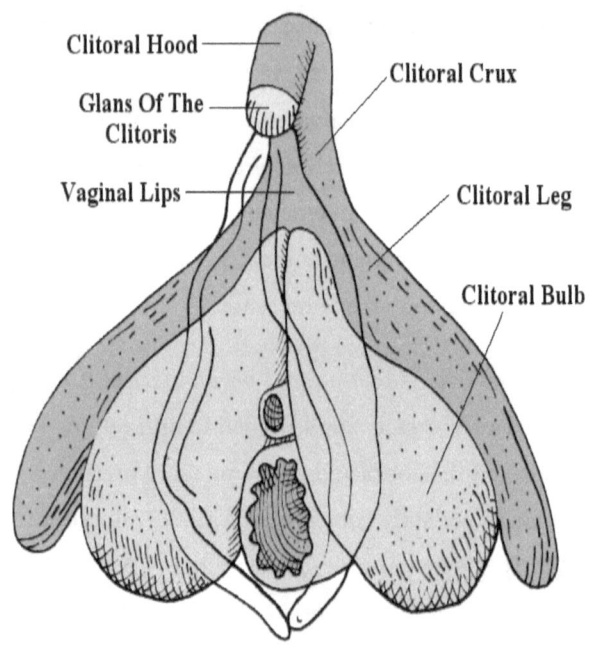

Clitoral Hood

Glans Of The
Clitoris

Vaginal Lips

Clitoral Crux

Clitoral Leg

Clitoral Bulb

Now I'm willing to bet that most of you have never seen an image like this one before. This is not an image of the vagina, the vulva or the female reproductive system. Those are the ones from sex ed. Flip ahead a few pages to see on like that, this one is different.

This one is, in fact, a diagram solely of the clitoris. As such, it's only a diagram that will help whoever is reading this book get and give more pleasure during sex. It's a diagram that will encourage you to have more sex and empower you to have better sex when you do. That, my friends, is exactly why they don't teach this in school. That's OK. I get it. Schools are not in the business of encouraging sex or teaching pleasure. They only want to teach the bare necessities, and even those belatedly. Understanding the clitoris and it's role in orgasm is not a bare necessity to sex and reproduction. It's a pleasurable luxury.

The problem is, that few people go back and figure this stuff out once they become responsible, normal sexually active and orgasm wanting adults. One of the aims of this book is to fix just that problem.

Enough ranting. Let's talk clitoris.

At the top of the above image, you'll see, clearly marked, the glans of the clitoris. This is what most people think of when they think clitoris. This is a tiny protrusion of highly sensitive tissue located just above the union of the two inner vaginal lips. This is what everybody is aiming for when there is any fingering, oral sex or vibrator play. That actually makes total sense, because this little area contains an amazingly high number of nerves and is the most sensitive spot on a woman's body. The glans, or the tip of the penis, is the same way in men. Stimulating the glans of the clitoris is no doubt capable of producing orgasms as any woman who has explored her body will attest.

But there's much, much more.

The clitoris doesn't stop with the glans. It is only the tip of much more. The tissue actually extends back into the woman's body quite a bit, then splits off to form two wishbone like legs that run down either side of the vulva. The place where the legs split off from the whole structure is called the clitoral crux and the legs are called the clitoral legs. This whole structure is made up of a material called corpus cavernosum.

I'm going to pause for a moment and talk about corpus cavernosum. Unless you're a doctor or an anatomist, I will forgive you for not recognizing what that is. Corpus cavernosum is a fancy Latin name for spongy tissue that can fill with blood and swell. It's also highly sensitive tissue loaded with nerves. Corpus cavernosum, for reference, is the exact same tissue that is in two of the three erectile structures in the shaft of the penis that fills with blood, enlarges the penis and allows it to get hard in preparation for intercourse. For the rest of this discussion, I am going to dispense with the term "corpus cavernosum" and replace it with "erectile tissue".

Just like the erectile tissue in the penis, the erectile tissue of the clitoral legs and crux both swell and enlarge when a woman is aroused. Note that. It's important.

There's still more clitoris though.

Beyond just the legs and the crux of the clitoris, there are two other structures of erectile tissue that you may not be familiar with. These are called the clitoral bulbs. The clitoral bulbs are also made up of erectile tissue, however, of a different type than the legs of the clitoris. These structures are made up of tissue known as corpus spongiosum. Corpus spongiosum, just like corpus cavernosum, fills with blood during arousal, swells and is loaded with nerves.

Corpus cavernosum makes up two of the three pockets of erectile tissue in the penis, like I mentioned a moment ago. Corpus spongiosum makes up the third. I want you to note that both the penis and the clitoris have three pockets of erectile tissue, two of corpus cavernosum and one of corpus spongiosum. That is both not an accident or a coincidence and we will talk about why that is as we progress through this chapter.

So, there is a lot more to the clitoris that they taught you in school. So what?

This fact actually has several implications that we needs to take note of.

The first is the fact that when most people think of and attempt to stimulate the clitoris, they are actually focusing on an area that is a tiny fraction of its full size. There's so much attention on that sensitive little nub we call the glans, that most people completely overlook the rest.

Think of it this way. How would men feel if the majority of women didn't even realize that there was any penis beyond the head? All they did was focus on the head and nothing else. It would take a lot of the depth and a lot of fun sexual activities. Blowjobs, to start, would be less effective, pleasurable and a lo more frustrating. That's for sure. By becoming aware of how much larger and complex the clitoris is, we afford ourselves the opportunity to stimulate the entire organ instead of just a tiny fraction of it. This allows for deeper, more complete arousal of the organ and much more powerful and pleasurable orgasms too.

Beyond just deeper arousal and more powerful orgasms, a

total knowledge of the anatomy clitoris is useful because it offers lovers the chance to introduce orgasms during intercourse to their love life. How is this possible?

Here's something else they didn't tell you in sex ed. Not only is the clitoris larger and more complex than you ever dared dream, but beyond that, all of the new parts that I just described to you are capable or producing an orgasm in a woman, in my opinion. Additionally, while the glans of the clitoris is not necessarily accessible during many intercourse positions, there are ways to stimulate the internal parts that I just introduced you to, and in many cases, from my experience, this stimulation can result in orgasm.

Throughout this chapter I'm going to talk about the misunderstood and under appreciated clitoris and we'll even bring the penis into the discussion, but first, I am going to give you some homework. This exercise will allow you (and your partner if you have one) to explore stimulating the internal clitoral structures. I'm a big fan of "seeing is believing". Put this book down, give it a try and come back when you've finished and you're ready to learn some more. I'm sure I'll have your undivided attention by that time.

Seeing Is Believing: Part A

It's always been my experience that nothing convinces someone that what you are saying is true like a demonstration that they can see with their own eyes. There is no reason to change that type of thinking at this point, so I will give you just such a demonstration.

We've discussed the internal structures of the clitoris. Now it's time to do a little exploring and see if you can't stimulate the parts I just described to you. There are two ways that this can be done. The first is by the woman on her own and the second is a couple doing some exploration together. Either one works, although there are variations depending on whether it's solo or tandem.

I will start first with the tandem. This is by no means a preference for the tandem act. Actually, I would recommend that any woman reading this do a little exploration on her own first and only after involve her partner This will make things a little easier. This way, she can guide him/her and show them what she's found. Plus, I believe that she'd be more comfortable without the immediate prying eyes of a lover. I'm writing about tandem first, because it will be a little easier to visualize if I write about two people, and from this, a woman on her own will be able to extrapolate and understand the solo part more easily.

To start with the tandem exercise, the woman should lie down on the bed. Set the mood. She should be very comfortable. There should be lots of pillows and make sure that the room is warm enough for nudity. Hiding under blankets from the cold is very much detrimental to this exercise. Don't forget soft lighting too. We don't want or need any cold fluorescent lights. Candlelight is good. Soft music is good too.

Next, she should bend her knees and spread her legs as wide as it's comfortable. She should let her knees drop open and spread naturally. Now, her partner is to sit between her legs in a cross legged fashion. Partners, I need to remind you that this is an intimacy building, body exploration. As hot, lovely and seductive as you find your partner to be, put a pin in that for now and focus on the exercise. What you learn here could really help with trust and more pleasurable sex down the road, so focus.

The aim of this exercise is to stimulate the internal parts of her clitoris. You are going to completely ignore the glans of the clitoris at this point, and instead you're only going to focus on the internal clitoris. Men, to make this a little more clear, this is going to be like her giving you a handjob in which she completely ignores the tip of your penis, but instead focuses on the shaft alone.

Start by placing the palm side of your fingers on either side of her vulva like it's shown in the above picture. At first, just let them lay there. This will allow her to get used to the warmth of your hands. It will begin physical arousal. It will also allow her body to begin to wake up to the idea that you are touching it. She would not just grab hold of your limp cock and start madly stroking and you should accord her pussy the same consideration. Let her warm up a little bit. Remember, her clitoris fills with blood and swells just like his penis and takes a little time. Don't be afraid to compliment her at this point either. She's feeling vulnerable and exposed. Tell her sincerely how beautiful she is.

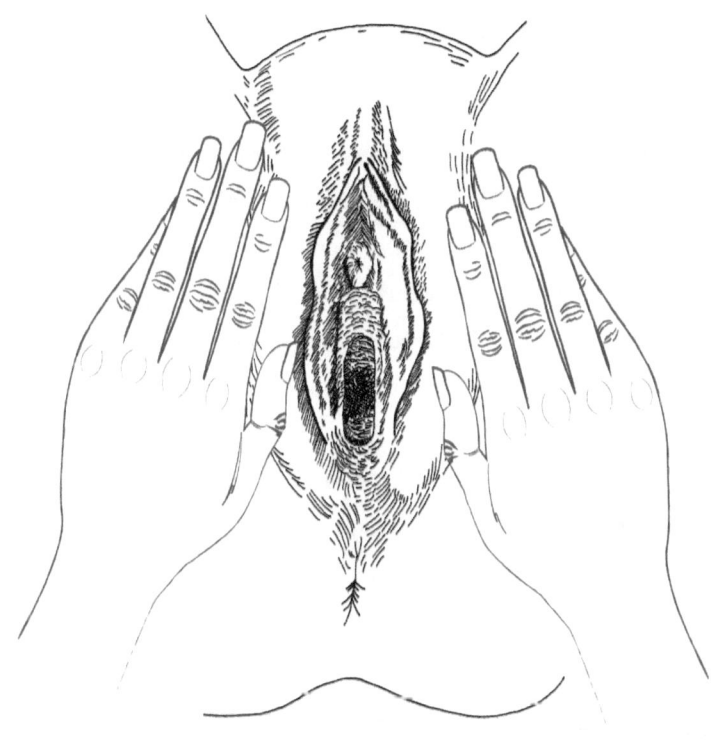

Once she's warmed up a little and is more responsive to your touch, you need to apply pressure INTO her pussy. If you are unclear on what I mean, lay your fingers flat on a table and them press down with them. This is what we're looking for. Start slow. Too little is better than too much and you can slowly apply more pressure. As you do, slowly begin to move your hands up and down. You're not rubbing her pussy, you're just moving your hands up and down and you're using the friction from the skin on skin contact to move her whole vulva up and down with them.

Remember, you are doing nothing to her external clitoris or her vagina. Instead, you have your hands placed on the outside of her pussy, specifically on her labia majora and you're moving her whole pussy around while gently applying pressure. Feel free to move around and experiment. Try up (towards the glans of her clitoris) and then down (towards her anus) and then moving your hands in a circular motion as well. Move slowly and gently and just let the friction move the skin around. As you do this you will be stimulating the crux of the clitoris as well as her clitoral bulbs.

Now while all of this is happening, whoever is doing the hands part needs to keep a low profile. Keep eye contact with her, but keep questions to a minimum. Just watch her and see what happens. You're exploring together. Ladies, help your partners out. Talk about what you're feeling and feel free to tell them what to do. Partners, when she gives you instructions, follow them. Remember, you're in this together and that means teamwork.

Now, if you are planning on doing a this exercise solo we

only need to make some small modifications. Instead of lying flat, I would recommend leaning against a supportive pile of pillows. One of those pillows people use to read in bed will work perfectly. We want you somewhere between lying flat and sitting straight up is best. This will allow a good range of movement with your hands. Spread your legs as wide as you can, comfortably, and let the muscles relax to the side as you do so.

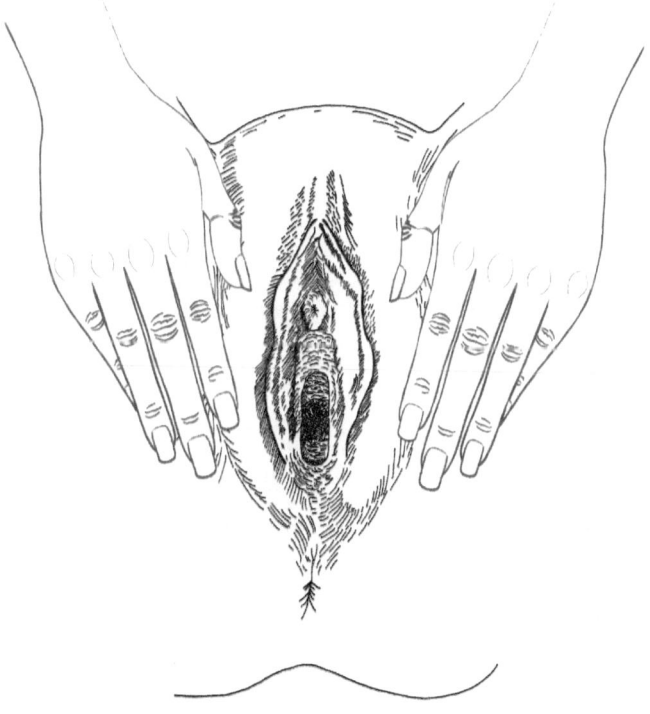

Then, slide your hands down on either side of your vulva and gently press inward with the flats of your fingers into yourself, just like in the picture below. Let them lay there. Let your pussy warm up to their touch, the same as with your lover. Give your clitoris a minute to get excited before you dive into the deep end of the pool. When you're ready, apply subtle, consistent pressure, just like in the tandem version. Slowly start moving the skin up and down using the friction of your hands.

Focus on the sides of your vulva, on the outer vaginal lips. Remember, the legs of the clitoris run under this skin and are very sensitive. We're looking to stimulate them with your touch. Move your hands up and down, and in circular motions. Try slow. See how it feels. Speed up. Increase and decrease pressure. What are you feeling?

Another trick you can try as you do this is you can move your hands closer together and sort of pinch your inner vaginal lips together with your outer lips. This will raise your vulva between your hands and will allow even more opportunities for pleasant stimulation. Take it nice and slow. Up and down works great in this situation. Remember to take your time. Close your eyes and relax your head and pay attention to the sensations and feelings in your body.

Now Let's Talk About The Penis

To many of you, it may seem odd for me to focus on the penis in a book that's all about the G-spot, the clitoris and how women orgasm. It's not really. The penis and the clitoris are very, very similar organs. No, they're not the same, but they do behave in very similar ways. Looking at one, is a lot like looking at your reflection in the mirror. Things are a little backwards but you get the idea of what is going on and the reflection will help you to better understand reality. The penis is the reflection of the clitoris and will help me to convince you of some more pretty cool similarities and possibilities. It'll also allow you to look at the idea that a large part of the penis is internal as well, just like the clitoris.

First, let's talk about how a baby's penis is formed before he's born. This, might seem a little off topic, but this is actually really important and shows where the similarities between the penis and the clitoris come from.

Early in a baby's development, like I've said before, you can't tell the sex. The DNA is set, but the physical characteristics don't necessarily reflect it. Up to a certain point, all babies, whether male or female, develop along the same path. Then, we come to a fork in the road. If a baby is male, some modifications of already formed tissue occur. To be blunt, what would form into a clitoris in a female baby changes into a penis.

Reflect back to the diagram of the internal clitoris that I already showed you. Now, use your imagination and follow along as I describe the process.

Imagine the glans of the clitoris growing outward and the clitoral legs growing out with it. The bulbs join together, extend out and wind up wrapping the urethra as it too grows longer. Now add skin, some nerves and some arteries to this and you have a penis. This whole, and I might add, vastly oversimplified process, leaves three separate shafts of erectile tissue inside the shaft of the penis. The glans of the penis is also still covered with a layer of retractable skin just like the glans of the clitoris is in women.

If you look at a cross section diagram of a penis, you can see the three separate and distinct pockets of erectile tissue that fill with blood and cause erections in sexually mature men.

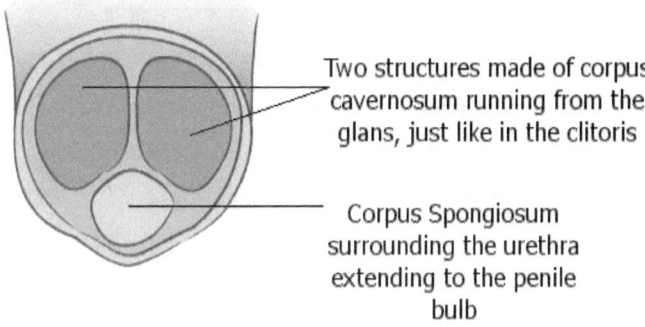

Two structures made of corpus cavernosum running from the glans, just like in the clitoris

Corpus Spongiosum surrounding the urethra extending to the penile bulb

These are essentially extensions of the same tissue structures that are present in a woman's clitoris. Yes, they are bigger and there are some added complexities, but by and large, the structures are very similar. In both the penis and the clitoris there are three separate pockets of erectile tissue. Two are made of corpus cavernosum and one is made of corpus spongiosum. Their places in the body are the same, more or less. The legs of the penis and the legs of the clitoris are both loaded with nerves, highly sensitive and swell during physical arousal. The same relationship is true of the clitoral bulbs and the singular penile bulb. They are located in similar spots, swell with blood and are very sensitive to stimulation. In biology, this similarity is called "analogous". This basically means, one thing performs a lot like another.

There is another analogous function that both penises and clitorises have. Both, upon stimulation are capable of producing orgasms that are very pleasurable. We'll talk more about that later, but for now, I just want you to understand that both penises and clitorises cause orgasms. This should be something we can all agree on.

Just like the clitoris, much of the penis is internal. The penis itself is external to the body, as I'm sure we've all seen. However, the full structure of the penis goes back into the body farther than you might imagine, just like the clitoris.

Looking at the following diagram, I would like you to take note of two structures in particular. The first is the penile leg that runs along the top portion of the shaft of the penis. This, if you are viewing this in color, is red. Keep in mind that this is one of two (refer back to the cross sectional diagram to get a better visual) and the other leg runs parallel to the visible one just behind it. Below, the legs of the penis, please note the blue erectile tissue that extends from the bulb of the penis, behind the scrotum, and runs all the way along the bottom side of the shaft to the glans (tip) of the penis.

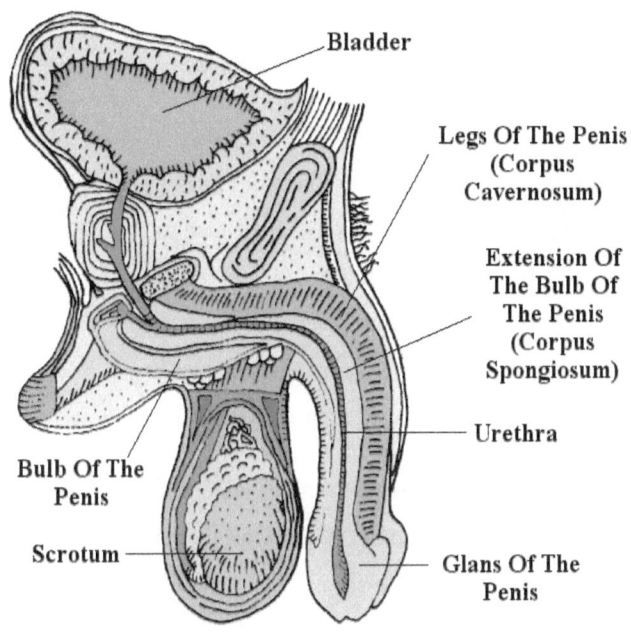

Bladder

Legs Of The Penis
(Corpus
Cavernosum)

Extension Of
The Bulb Of
The Penis
(Corpus
Spongiosum)

Urethra

Bulb Of The
Penis

Scrotum

Glans Of The
Penis

Why is all of this important?

Here's why.

I have shown you that the penis and the clitoris are very similar in character. The penis is literally made from the clitoris, and as such, shares many of its attributes. Both penises and clitorises have two legs of erectile tissue as well as bulbs. In the penis it's one joined bulb, in the clitoris it's two unjoined ones. Both structures swell with blood and become engorged during physical arousal. Both are also loaded with nerves, that upon stimulation, result in pleasurable orgasms.

If you stimulate the head, or glans of a man's penis that is the most sensitive, you will quickly be able to make him cum. This happens all the time during fellatio. The same thing happens during cunnilingus with a woman. Her lover puts their mouth on the glans (again, the external tip of the clitoris) and she will often orgasm quickly.

But, did you know that you can stimulate the erectile tissue of a man's penis, ignoring the glans all together and still give him an orgasm? You can. This part of the body is less sensitive than the glans. It will usually take longer for this reason, but you can definitely make him cum. Additionally, stimulating the penis while ignoring the glans will often result in more powerful, more intense orgasms. How interesting.

The penis is made from the clitoris. The penis and the clitoris behave very similarly. Much of the clitoris is internal. Much of the penis is internal. The penis fills with blood and swells during arousal. The clitoris fills with blood and swells during arousal. The clitoris is highly sensitive. The penis is highly sensitive. Stimulation of the glans of the penis results in orgasm. Stimulation of the glans of the clitoris results in orgasm.

Clearly, there are many physiological similarities.

If we can give a man a slower, more powerful orgasm by stimulating only the legs and the bulb of the penis, why can't a woman cum by stimulating the legs and the bulbs of her clitoris.

Now here's my conjecture. Interestingly enough, I believe she can, from my own personal experiences and empirical research.

By stimulating the internal and less sensitive parts of a woman's clitoris, it's likely you can give her an orgasm. Just like a man, it's usually slower, more powerful and it helps if there is lots of kissing and mental arousal to go with it, but I do believe it's possible.

More interestingly, while the glans of the clitoris is often a little tricky to stimulate during intercourse, with the exception of manual stimulation during sex from behind, it's actually pretty easy to stimulate the internal parts of the clitoris. That is to say, once you know where they are and are willing to make the effort.

In the rest of this book, I plan to show you how to experiment with and discover how to do just that whether you are a woman, a man or a couple. They didn't teach you this in school, but everyone should definitely know this stuff.

Seeing Is Believing: Part B

It's time that for the second part of my "Seeing Is Believing" exercise series. This one focuses on the penis. This exercise can be done solely by a man or as a couple. It's best done as a couple as it will afford you both an opportunity to see that this does work as well as creating a bonding moment, intimacy and some mutual discovery and more open communication. The open communication will be especially helpful later if you choose to try the rest of what this book will teach you.

In this exercise, we are going to give a handjob, but it's going to be a little different than normal. When most men masturbate, they seem to use lubrication and do a full stroke over the head of their penis. That's where we are going to differ. We're going to completely ignore the head and instead, do a much narrower stroke only over the shaft. Basically, stroke the penis from where it attaches to his body up to the start of the head and then go back down.

Don't use lubrication either. It will complicate things and make getting the exact stroke length a little harder. Instead, firmly grip the shaft and move the skin up and down over the erectile tissue like you did in the last exercise with her. Don't move your hand against the skin, move the skin over the shaft with your hand. Without lubrication, this should be fairly easy and chaffing shouldn't be an issue. Penises are built to be used a little roughly. In many ways they're similar to a battering ram.

If you're doing this as a couple, this is the perfect time for lots and lots of kissing. This is a less sensitive part of his body, just like the internal parts of her clitoris are less sensitive. Stimulating either can result in an orgasm, but mental arousal will help a lot with both. Kissing is the perfect way to get his mind into the action. When that happens, he will relax, surrender to the moment, get lost in kisses, build his arousal and cum in due course. If you're solo, porn will be a poorer substitute, but it will work in pretty much the same way.

Now take your time.

This part of the penis, like I've said, is less sensitive and it will take longer to build an orgasm. Slow, steady, consistent stimulation is what we are looking for. Be patient. Let it happen. She will need to let it happen when it comes time to stimulate the internal parts of her clitoris. This is also a great exercise to teach patience and empathy. When the two of you are working together to give her an orgasm, he will understand better, because he's sort of been there and done that.

Most likely, he will cum eventually as long as you keep the stimulation, slow, steady and consistent.

When you as a couple or you alone finally do orgasm using this technique, you may notice something else. You (the man) will notice that the orgasm is usually a lot stronger than normal. This should not come as a surprise since it most likely took longer to build. We'll talk more about that shortly. It's relevant, but note it for now.

Whether you do this as a couple or solo, I would strongly encourage you to take some time to talk about this experience as a couple, if applicable. What was it like? How did it feel? What did you like? Dislike? His experiences can help her understand her own, build confidence, create common understanding and shared perceptions. All of these will be very useful when you as a couple explore stimulating her internal clitoris together.

Remember, penises and clitorises are very similar and what applies to one often applies to both.

For Me, The Simple, Obvious Explanation

And now we come to the heart of the matter.

I don't, like I have said repeatedly in this book, believe in the G-Spot. For me, there's just too little evidence. It doesn't make any sense either. Why would women have two means of orgasming and men only have one? Remember, the male body is made, during embryo formation, from the female body. So it would make sense, logically speaking, if a woman had two organs that could give her an orgasm, than a man should too. But, according to all the men I have ever met, they only have one.

What if there was a much simpler and obvious explanation? Of course, I think you already know where I am going with this.

What if there was no G-Spot, but instead, all of these instances where women orgasm during sex, as a result of intercourse, were nothing more than a clitoral orgasm brought about by the stimulation of her internal clitoral parts through the front wall of the vagina?

That's what I believe to be the case.

We all believe that stimulating the clitoris will give a woman an orgasm. I've shown you how the clitoris is larger than most people think and how all of it's parts are made up of the same erectile tissue that makes up the penis. I have shown you how a penis can be made to orgasm by only stimulating the same erectile tissue that makes up the body of the clitoris. What I have not shown you is how the clitoris could very easily play the part of the G-Spot given its actual size and its orientation in a woman's body. In essence, I believe, the mysterious G-Spot gets all the credit, when in reality, it is the clitoris that's doing all the work.

Recall back to the beginning of this book when I talked about the origin of the "G-Spot" with Grafenburg's description. He mentioned a spot of sensitivity on the front wall of the vagina, running parallel to the urethra. To paraphrase, stimulating a woman's vagina along the front wall, along the line of the urethra gave women orgasms.

Please refer back to the diagram of the internal clitoris and note the location of the urethra, vagina and clitoral crux.

Are we all on the same page?

Look at the following diagram to see the same spatial

orientation from a different perspective.

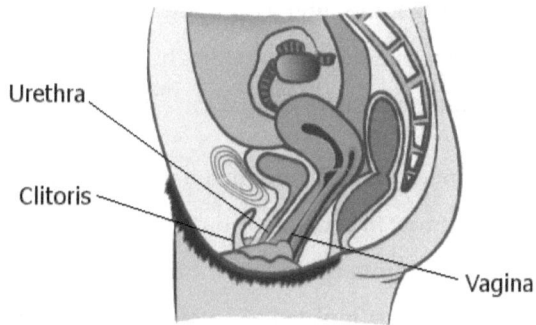

(Keep in mind, while looking at the above image, that the legs of the clitoris come down from the marked spot and lie on both sides of the vaginal and urethral openings.)

If you look, you will see clearly labeled, the vagina, the urethra and the clitoris. Look at their arrangement in the diagram. Now, imagine inserting a finger into this woman's vagina and imagine pressing is along the front wall (the front side of her body where her belly button is). If you did this, you would see that you were applying pressure to tissue that contained her urethra, just like Grafenburg said, but you would also be applying pressure to the back of the body of her internal clitoris.

Rather than believing that there is some mysterious spot in a woman's urinary system that causes orgasm, to me, it is much, much easier to believe that while doing this, I am stimulating the larger, hidden, internal parts of her clitoris. No one disputes that the clitoris can cause orgasms and its close proximity to the very spot that has been suggested to be the location of the elusive G-Spot can't be overlooked.

Candidly, it's much easier for me, and hopefully you, to believe that at times, in certain positions, a woman's clitoris is being stimulated from behind, or the legs and bulbs of the clitoris are being stimulated to cause an orgasm rather than to believe in some organ that can't even be definitively located by modern medical science.

It all boils down to basic common sense for me. This isn't a question of belief. There is no faith at issue here. This is science and reason. The clitoris is real. It's tangible. It's existence is not disputed. Plus, it's right there where the G-Spot is supposed to be and, with a little effort, can be stimulated during sex. Occam's razor still holds true in this day and age. That is, the simplest explanation is usually the correct one. For me, in my opinion, the large and internal clitoris is a much simpler and reasonable explanation for where a woman's orgasm during sex derives.

Positions & Orgasms During Sex - Reinforcing This Point

My asking around and empirical research has suggested to

me that it's more common for women who can orgasm during sex, to do so when they're in the top position. This, is a very useful bit of information to us in our pursuit of the truth.

Why would this be the case? Why would a woman, now that you know what you do about the extensive nature of the clitoris be more likely to orgasm when she is in the top position?

The answer has three parts, as I see it.

The first part of this answer is flush contact. Flush contact is the pressing of her entire vulva against her lover's body. The glans of her clit usually gets left out but her labia majora and the clitoral legs beneath don't. Flush contact with her vulva means the internal clitoris is being stimulated. All of that engorged erectile tissue is getting stimulated.

During "him on top" positions, this is not always guaranteed. It depends a lot on where his weight is, how he is entering her and depth of penetration. Plus, when he pulls back out with each stroke, flush contact is broken. This makes the stimulation intermittent when he is on top, at best.

This is not true when she is on top in say, the cowgirl position. She is on top of him, straddling him and facing him. In this position, her entire vulva will be pressed into him the entire time he is inside of her. Body to body contact will be there 100% of the time while the couple is making love. Plus, 100% of the time, all of the internal parts of her clitoris will get stimulation. This is the perfect way to create the same sensations you and her discovered in "Seeing Is Believing: Part A" however, everybody's hands are free for other activity. The bodies pressing together, plus hip movement will do all the work automatically.

Control is another essential element that's present when she is on top. This raises the chances of her experiencing an orgasm during intercourse. When he is on top, he is in control of the action. He moves in response to his pleasure. I'm not saying men are inconsiderate or anything like that. I'm just saying that he's not in tune with her pleasure like when she's on top.

When the woman is on top, she can move her whole body and control what happens. Using her hips and thighs, she can rub up and grind where it feels good. She can pull back and use the shaft of his penis to create all kinds of pleasant stimulation to all the parts of her clitoris. This ability is completely absent when he is on top. It just won't happen.

Consistency is the last element that's missing when the man's on top that's present when the woman's on top.

When he's on top and he's entering her, he is usually all over the map. He might move in a way or rub up on something that feels great for a moment or two, but more often than not, he moves away after that. When a woman is on top, this isn't a problem. She can move where she wants it, rub and grind as she pleases and keep it up as long as she wants. The tails are turned when she's on top and she's moving in harmony with her pleasure.

Stop and think about all of that When a woman is on top, she is in a better body position to directly stimulate her internal clitoris, just like we did in "Seeing Is Believing: Part A". In addition to that, she can move and adjust to how things feel best to her. Lastly, she can keep that up as long as she likes, because she is in control of the action.

If I'm right about the internal clitoris being responsible for women cumming during sex, not the G-Spot, then all three of the differences that I just listed would make it much more likely for women to cum when they are on top during sex. That is precisely what I've found to be the case during conversations with women in my life.

Popular Vibrators Add Credit To The Explanation

When I was growing up, the best vibrator you could get was a either a plug into the wall model you bought in the "beauty" section of the grocery store or a basic slimline model. The slimline, phallic ones were harder to come by. Most women would buy them mail order so they didn't have to go into a "dirty bookshop". As a result, most women that I knew had the ones from the beauty section. You probably know they type. Big white vibrating head on it, you plug it into the wall and then press the whole vibrating head into your vulva.

You really had to be careful that you just didn't shoot past and orgasm as the thing rattled your teeth.

That was then. This is now and vibrators have come a long way. The more popular ones lend a lot of credit to the common sense theory I'm advocating in this book. Let's talk about that.

Ask almost any woman and she'll tell you that the best type of vibrator to buy is a rabbit style vibrator. This is a phallic shaped vibrator that is about 7" long covered in silicone rubber. The shaft of the silicone penis vibrates. There's more though.

In addition to the vibrating silicone cock, there is a part on the battery housing that curves around and presses firmly against the glans of the clitoris. Usually it's shaped like some kind of cute cuddly animal. Just what you want on your sensitive bits. But wait. There's still more. The shaft of the silicone penis is filled with balls that rotate inside your vagina adding even more stimulation.

Taken all together, there are a lot of fun, vibrating, moving parts to bring on quick and powerful orgasms.

But why are those orgasms so quick and powerful?

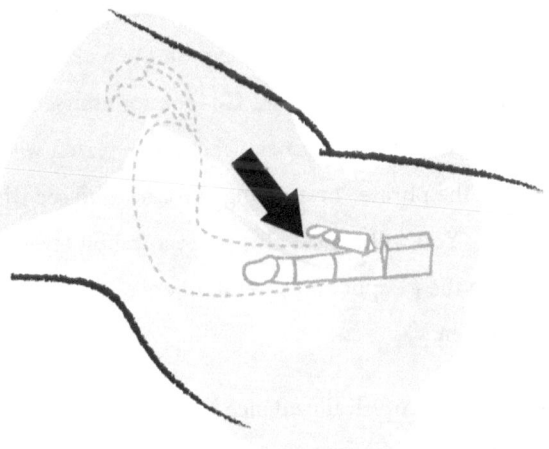

With a rabbit style vibrator, the clitoris is held between the glans stimulating portion and the the vibrating shaft as shown by the arrow in the above image. This provides both internal and external stimulation simultaneously.

In the context of all the information I have given you about the internal structure and the actual size and shape of the clitoris, it isn't hard to tell. These toys are stimulating the glans of the clitoris at the same time they are stimulating the crux and bulbs of the clitoris from the inside of the vagina through the front wall. Add to that that the woman has a nice silicone cock to grip down on and you have a powerful combination. Literally, all the parts of her clitoris are getting powerful stimulation from every direction. Her vagina is filled as well. Think 360° of stimulation. Small surprise the orgasms are so quick and powerful.

It's not hard to understand why this particular type of sex toy is one of the most popular types on the market today but, don't take my word for it. Go look for yourself. Find a sex toy retailer on the internet. Then, do a search with their name and the phrase "best selling vibrator" and see what comes up. You will almost always see a "rabbit style" vibrator in the #1 spot and several others of the same style in the top ten.

That is strong empirical evidence of women voting with their dollars. No, it's not 100% scientific, but it certainly suggests things to us. It suggests to me that women are buying vibrators to stimulate their clitorises internally and externally simultaneously.

To me, that was just more evidence that I was right to dismiss the G-Spot and focus on the clitoris.

How The Simple Explanation Explains The Large Variety Of Orgasm Experiences

It's no secret that women have a large variety of experiences when it comes to orgasms during sex. Most just don't cum during sex. Some do infrequently. Some come close a lot. A minority would tell you they cum during sex routinely. Why are there so many different experiences and how does the simple explanation that the clitoris is responsible for all of a woman's orgasms explain it?

I believe there's a simple, logical explanation for this question too.

We all take it for granted that there are a lot of different penises out there. There are growers. There are showers. Some are bigger than others. Some are too big. Some are just right. Some curve to the left. Some to the right. Some...well, you get the point. There are lots and lots of different penises out there. In fact, while they share many common elements and there are lots of similarities to how they like to be touched, it's fairly safe to say that no two penises are alike.

So why would we assume that one clitoris is exactly like another? I don't think we should.

Here's some more logic. If we all agree that no two penises are exactly alike, and we also agree that penises are formed from clitorises before birth, it would seem logical that clitorises would be as varied as penises. Wouldn't they?

Every clitoris is different. Every one will enjoy being stimulated slightly differently from any one else. Locations may vary. Locations may vary a lot. Size may vary a lot too. One woman may have a larger clitoris that extends farther into her body than another and offers more opportunity for stimulation. There may be less tissue between one woman's vaginal wall and the crux of her clitoris than another. Sensitivity may vary. Every woman, just like every man is made just a little differently.

However, that in itself, offers an explanation to the many different experiences women have concerning orgasms during sex. Most penises fall within a certain size range – an average really. Condom manufacturers size their condoms according to this average. Well, clitorises, it would seem have an average too. Most women would seem to fall into this category. This, I would argue is the category that has trouble orgasming spontaneously (that is without intentional stimulation) during sex. The women who can cum spontaneously during sex, without having to make an effort, are outside of this average group. Candidly, they're just the lucky ones, but my empirical research suggests they're in the minority.

Now don't go and hang your head. What I'll call an average woman, who does not spontaneously orgasm during sex, can most definitely stimulate their clitoris during sex, can most definitely add to her pleasure during sex, and with a good partner, some patience and some focus, can possibly orgasm during sex as well. We'll talk about that very shortly.

Intercourse Orgasms Are Often Reported To Feel Better. Why?

In putting this little book together, I spoke to lots of women about their experiences with orgasm. We had lots of frank discussions and, added to my own experiences, this empirical body of evidence began to offer insights and trends. One of the trends that I noticed was that many women who say they do experience orgasms during sex, say that the orgasms are more intense. This agrees with my own experiences as well.

I have, up to this point, expressed my belief that all orgasms come from the clitoris and there's no such thing as the G-Spot. Yet, now, I am pointing out that there are differences in the orgasms produced. This is something that I need to explain if I hope to convince you that my conjecture is correct.

I will assume that all of my readers, male or female, have had an orgasm at some point. If that's true, it should not come as a surprise that I'm asserting that not all orgasms are the same. There are great orgasms. There are bad orgasms. There are in between orgasms. The orgasms that you have when you masturbate are much lower in quality than those at the end of a night of marathon lovemaking with a partner you find incredibly attractive and have wanted since you first laid eyes on them. If orgasms were coffee, one would be old gas station coffee that's been in the pot all day and the other is a freshly ground and brewed exquisite cup of Italian espresso. Both are coffee, but there are obvious, palpable differences.

If we can agree that there's a natural range of orgasm potency, it should be a little easier to show you why and how orgasms produced by stimulating the internal clitoris are often "more powerful" than other orgasms.

Like the penis, the majority of nerves in the clitoris are

located in the glans at the very tip. However, also like the penis, the rest of the organ does have nerves, is still quite sensitive and is ultimately, in my opinion, is capable of producing an orgasm. However, just like stroking the shaft of the penis only, the process of getting there is slower than if the glans itself were stimulated.

During intercourse, as the internal parts of the clitoris are being stimulated, the building towards orgasm is a lot slower and more drawn out because the tissue is much less sensitive than at the glans. That allows the mental arousal to heighten and build at the same time the physical arousal moves along towards a crescendo. The longer the anticipation and the build up, the more powerful the release when it finally happens, generally speaking.

Thinking about it another way might make it a little easier to convince you before I move on to another topic.
Imagine, man or woman, that today is a special day for you.
Your lover is giving you a gift. Every hour today, they will give you oral sex for two minutes. It won't be enough to cum, but it will be a lot of fun, then, at midnight, they'll give you oral sex until you cum. With me so far?

I think it would be fairly easy for all of us to agree that when you finally do cum, it will be very intense. There will have been hour after hour of anticipation, mental arousal and physical stimulation. You'll be wound so tight, you may not even be able to cum at that point. Your body will be one big hair triggered tangle of nerves and impulses. But, if you do cum, we should all agree, the orgasm will be Earth shattering and may scramble your brains.

Orgasms during intercourse, if and when they do happen, often take longer to achieve and, as a result, even though they are still clitoral orgasm in my opinion, are much more powerful and pleasurable. Stimulating the internal parts of the clitoris allows enough time for a woman's mind and body to work together to create a much more intense release. But the bottom line is they still originate with her clitoris.

Admitting I Wasn't Supposed To Cum During Sex Freed Me To Do Just That

I know I keep liberally applying personal experience into this narrative. Well, I'm the author and that's my prerogative. So here's another one that I think many of my readers might find useful.

While sitting in that same bean bag chair where I reasoned out just how unnecessary my orgasm was to my "basic role in biology", I had another epiphany that wound up being really useful to me. I concluded, that if my orgasm was unnecessary, which I still believed (more so even), than it wasn't a huge leap to conclude that I wasn't supposed to cum during sex. If it did happen, it was more of an accident than anything else. Basically, if it happened, my clitoris had sort of accidentally gone off.

Like I said, that was huge for me. I'd been wondering if there was something wrong with me. I'd been wondering all this time if I had been having sex wrong. The conclusion that I wasn't "supposed" to cum during sex freed me from both of these issues. No, I had been having sex right and there was nothing wrong with me. Instead of trying to unravel the impossible knot, I just cut the rope.

What I realized, was that in order to orgasm during sex, which Mother Nature never intended, I was going to need to have sex in ways that Mother Nature hadn't planned on either.

I don't mean anything like anal. Don't worry.

Here's what I mean. When animals have sex, it's brief, functional, purpose driven and to the point. The positions are basic, usually doggystyle regardless of the animal. Humans and chimpanzees are the only known animals to do it face to face. It's usually short and then it's done. It's all about completion and little to nothing about her pleasure.

In order to cum during sex, I needed sex to be drawn out and longer than normal. I needed to transform sex from functional and purpose driven to recreational, hedonistic encounters that were marathon sessions in lieu of brief encounters. I needed to take sex to a higher level. Just like making him cum without touching the glans of his penis, a clitoral orgasm during sex takes time to build. I needed to find positions that stimulated all the parts of my clitoris during sex. After I found them, I reasoned, I would need to communicate and work with my partner to keep the stimulation consistent enough to let my orgasm build. We would have to work as a team, be truly intimate and connected with each other and be of one mind.

I did a lot of experimenting. I mean a lot of experimenting.

It turned out finding the positions was the easy part.

Clitoris Stimulating Positions – With Training Wheels

Now we've come to the part that I'm sure you're all interested in. This is the part where we talk about how to put everything that we've just learned to create opportunities for internal clitoris stimulation and maybe, just maybe, orgasms during sex.

This is some exciting stuff and I won't keep you waiting.

For anyone interested in applying what they have learned, I would recommend two and only two sexual positions to start with. Keeping it simple makes success more likely. The first is commonly referred to as the cowgirl position. Please take note that I said "cowgirl" and not "reverse cowgirl". The second is the classic missionary position.

I'm going to start with cowgirl. This is the natural place to start, as I have already spelled out the reasons that women would be, and seem to be more likely to cum in this position. However, now I'm going to provide you with a detailed, exploration exercise to help you get started.

Start by having him lie on the bed with his legs close together. Now, you straddle his bikini zone and take his penis and slip it inside of you. (I am assuming foreplay and that everyone is excited and ready to go, physically speaking, especially her. That means lots and lots of lube. We'll talk more about foreplay and its importance in the next chapter.)

Now, she's sitting on top of his pelvis and he's lying there.

Good. We're ready to begin.

The first thing I want to make sure that the couple understands is that we are not doing any thrusting. That is how normal sex goes. The man or woman makes his penis go in and out and after a short while, he's cumming and that's pretty much the end of things. That's not what we're doing here. Remember, we're having sex in ways Mother Nature did not plan on.

In this exercise, no one is doing an thrusting. For all intents and purposes, she's just going to hold his erect penis with her vagina and he's going to let her. He's going to hold still and let her move as much as she wants and where she wants while he is motionless. The only time that he should be moving is after she asks him to do so in a way that will help with her pleasure. Men, you'll need to be patient here. However, in the long run that patience will mean so much to her and a lot more sex for you. Keep that in mind. For the men, patience is the word of the day.

So she's sitting on top of his cock, holding it in her vagina and neither one of them is doing any in and out moving. Good. We're right where we want to be. The couple is physically connected. Now, we need to get them spiritually connected and feeling close, passionate and united. To do that, we kiss. We kiss a lot.

Kissing is the reason that cowgirl is the position I chose for this exercise, rather than reverse cowgirl. There is so much magic in kissing and we would be foolish to exclude it from this exercise. We can say volumes with our lips without ever uttering a word, and that's exactly what we are about to do.

She lowers her lips to his and the two, while still physically connected, join their lips and hopefully their passions, souls, goals and minds.

In addition to all the ethereal reasons I just mentioned to kiss, there are two very real and practical ones. The first is that she needs to be good and excited. Her physical arousal needs time to reach its peak before she can effectively begin to explore her internal clitoris and the kissing will do just that. Once her arousal is at its peak, her clitoris and its internal structures will be swelled with blood and much more sensitive. In addition, we want to make sure her vagina is very well lubricated. She will be sitting on his cock for a while and the lubrication will ensure her comfort. Lots of kissing means lots of lubrication, comfort and arousal.

We also want to make sure that he's very aroused too. His

cock might be a little confused by what's going on. Remember, this is different than normal. Chances are in his whole sexual life, he's never just stayed inside a woman without any thrusting. Honestly, it's unnatural and a little weird for a man, especially the first time. It goes against all of his instincts. When cocks get confused, they have a tendency to go limp and that's not what we need. We need him to be rock hard and very physically aroused for her to explore stimulating her internal clitoris. All this kissing, heavy breathing, closeness and intimacy will make sure that he stays hard, aroused and very eager.

The kissing should go on for a while. Just keep it going. He just lies there and kisses. That's his only job. Honestly, it will be helpful if his mind just went blank and his world was 100% about her kisses and nothing more. Very zen. He needs to show patience and allow her arousal to reach its peak. Look, I know she'll be excited and eager to explore. That's the nature of a woman learning how to orgasm. However, she needs to be patient too. Ladies, wait until you think you're ready. Then, wait and kiss some more.

It will be helpful if you can wait and draw out the kissing until you are a live wire of horniness and you feel if you don't get a chance to cum soon you'll just go crazy. When you get to this point, then you're ready to begin the next phase.

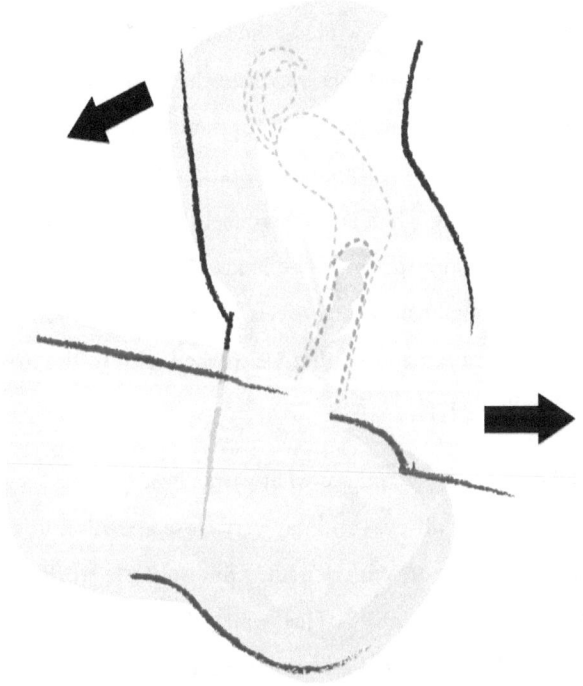

The next phase is actual stimulation of the internal (and yes, possibly external too) parts of the clitoris. This is much more personal. I don't mean that I won't talk about it. I mean that your clitoris is very different than mine and any other woman's in the world. Remember? We already talked about that already. Now, is when you figure out what works best for you and how to make yourself feel really good.

I will say that leaning forward helps a lot for me. Lean forward with your torso, while at the same time sliding your hips back. This will push his cock into the front wall of your vagina, which is where the clitoral crux is. That always feels really good. Beyond that, try rotating your hips in a circle and deciding when and where feels best. Moving my hips backwards and forwards, while keeping my vulva pressed firmly against his body feels really good too. This stimulates those same areas that we worked with in the first "Seeing Is Believing" exercise.

Give all of these a try and see what works best for you. Explore. Close your eyes and pay very close attention to all the sensations you are experiencing. Shut out the world and retreat into your mind. He'll wait. He'll hold still. Trust me. He's as excited and eager about this as you are and nothing in the world will make him as happy as you sitting on top of his still cock, slowly exploring your own pleasures and using his body like some sort of sexual jungle gym. That's on every man's fantasy wish list.

Men, while she's exploring, like I've said, hold your body still. Don't move your hips in anyway unless she tells you to. Be still and loving and let her explore. Don't ask questions. Don't offer encouragement. In fact, say nothing unless she asks you something. Be loving, patient and kind and let her explore. Trust me. She will be very, very thankful later. I'm sure. Also, if you start to feel that you are getting close to cumming, close your legs and press them together. That will help ward of an orgasm that would spoil this for both of you. Do this as many times as needed.

Also men, your hands should not be idle during all of this, but they shouldn't be busy either. Try laying them gently on her thighs. That way, she will feel connected to you, but you will not limit her movement as she explores or distract her. Avoid her hips and ass. Those shouldn't be impeded.

Alright ladies, back to you.

As you explore, you will find parts of your body held one way or another, will feel great. As you discover these spots, positions and sensations, you can begin to repeat them. Honestly, there are a lot of parallels here to when you first started exploring your body and accidentally discovered how to masturbate. It's the same for all of us and it's the same here.

"That feels good. Huh."

"I think I'll do that some more. Maybe harder. Maybe faster."

"Ooooh. That feels even better. Maybe harder. Maybe faster."

We all know how this story ended the first time and we may be able to repeat it with patience and practice. It's the same for women as it is for men and every person who has ever lived really. Wow. That feels great. I'll just keep doing it. Then...an orgasm sneaks up, our head is spinning, our thighs are twitching and powerful, pleasurable waves are running through our bodies. Before we know it, it's over, we're euphoric and we can't wait to do it again.

Girls, with you on top of your patient, silent men, it's no different. Explore. Find out what feels good. Try it another way. Maybe harder. Maybe faster. Your own clitoris will determine what works for you. If an orgasm comes on, great. If not, keep doing this as long as you like or as long as he can stand it. Every minute you do it feels great and teaches you more and more about your body, your pleasure, what you like and what feels great. For me, it took a fair amount of trying and experimenting before anything interesting ever happened. I just had to keep at it.

Additionally, the longer that this goes on, the more comfortable you will be, the more relaxed you'll be, the more aroused you'll be and the more likely you will be able to orgasm. The first time that my lover and I tried this, it lasted quite a long time. My thighs were exhausted at the end as the orgasm snuck up on me like a tiger in tall grass. However, when it did, all the building, connection, closeness, intimacy and arousal paid off in a way that I'll remember forever.

Cowgirl is really the best option because it allows the person who can feel the clitoral stimulation to direct the motion and the stimulation in a way that best pleases her. However, some women just don't like being on top and want to be on the bottom. It feels nice to have him on top of you with his weight comfortingly bearing down on you like a heavy blanket on a snowy night. I'd be lying if I said I didn't really enjoy that as he kisses me deeply. Sometimes you just need that feeling.

For those of you who want that sensation, while at the same time having your internal clitoris stimulated, I can offer your another option. I will say that this one's a lot harder and usually takes longer but it has worked for me in the past so I'll pass it on to you.

This exercise is based on the missionary position. She lies on her back, spreads her legs and he lies between them with his penis inside of her.

Just like in the last exercise, there should be lots and lots of kissing. All of the same reasons apply. We want her to be well lubricated and very aroused, the same as him. Also, again like the last time, there should be no thrusting in and out. That's not what we're looking for. That will only make him very excited and most likely lead to a quick, exercise ending orgasm.

He should put himself inside of her to his full length and just stay there, again, still, and then he should busy himself in kissing her. It's generally helpful if he rests his weight on his knee and forearms. He should not smother her with his weight and rest it all on her. That will only limit her range of motion for what comes next.

Lastly, he should push into her vagina with his pelvis and try to maintain the pressure as best he can. No in and out, just steady, inward pressure from his glutes and thighs that presses the root area of his cock flush against her vulva.

Then, with his cock still fully inside her, he lifts up with his thighs. This upward pressure will force the shaft of his penis into the front wall of her vagina. There, it can apply pressure to the back of her clitoral crux.

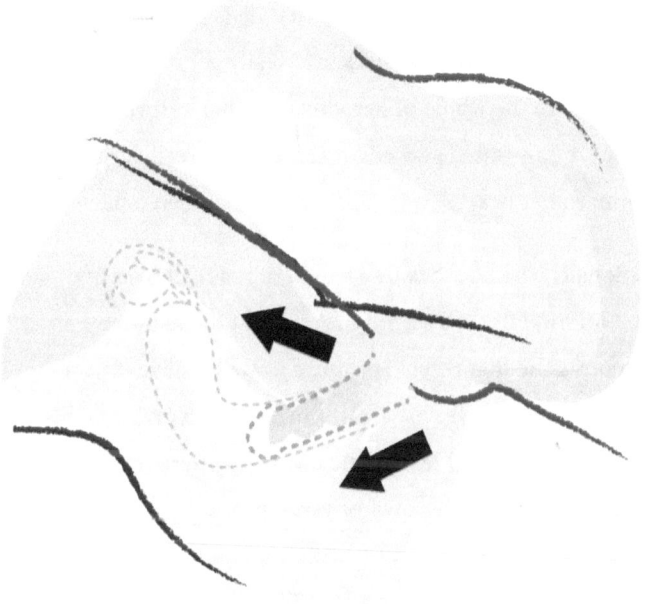

Once he is pressing into her with his pelvis, is up on his knees and is kissing her, she is free to repeat the exploration steps that he talked about with her on top. This is the exact same process, except she is doing it from a different angle and has two potential bonuses. She should try everything that I talked about before. Try pressing the front wall of your vagina with the clitoral crux against the shaft of his penis. Rotate your hips. Press up. Press down. Try it all, discover what you like, repeat, enhance, increase, go faster and see what happens.

The first advantage is the pressure that he is producing. This will allow her to press back and really get some good stimulation to the whole of her vulva. As her clitoris becomes fully aroused and engorged, she can really grind into him to her heart's content. For me, that feels amazing.

Additionally, she now has free hands to roam all over his body. All too often we seem to forget that the hands are an erogenous zone that receive pleasure as well as give it. She can run her hands over his arms, through his hair, along his neck, thighs, butt, and legs as she explores different positions to enhance her own physical pleasure. Add to that that she can grasp his hips with her hands to physically direct and control his movements. This combination of mental as well as physical stimulation and control can be very useful.

Both of these exercises have worked for me in my own sex life and my partner and I have learned how to achieve orgasm during both of these, working together. These will offer you a great place to get started with your lover. Try them out. See what you like and what works for you. As you become more self aware, you should try other positions and see how those work for you too and what advantages, benefits and challenges that they afford. For now though, stick to these, work together, and see where they lead you.

Helpful Intangibles

Finding the positions that stimulated my clitoris during sex was the easy part. We talked about those in the last chapter. Now, we come to the harder parts. There were other challenges. Communicating with my lover, being patient, keeping things in perspective, getting over my bashfulness and training my mind to believe orgasms during sex were possible were just some of the issues that cropped up.

Those, the intangible challenges and my experiences with them, are what this chapter is all about.

I will admit, this chapter is a bit of an eclectic one. There is no one central theme. The pieces of this chapter don't flow together in a fluid way like the last ones did. I can't show you exactly how to overcome these obstacles. Every woman/man/couple who reads this book will be faced with a unique combination at least some of these issues, I suspect. I don't have a one size fits all approach to these, but I knew that I needed to acknowledge all of these issues to better inform my readers.

How to do that preoccupied my mind for a bit. I couldn't figure out exactly how I wanted to tackle these. Then it hit me. Personal anecdotes and stories that illustrate the problems and pitfalls as well as the ways that my partner and I overcame them. The end result was this short and sweet little chapter full of personal tales and details.

If the rest of this book reads like some lost sex ed lesson from high school, it is my hope that this chapter reads more like an intimate conversation with a friend over coffee. It's my sincere hope that the very personal details I've included in this chapter will give you inspiration and ideas to overcome the same problems should they appear in your own life.

Tunnel Vision & Fun

When I first suspected that a woman's orgasm during sex was coming from her clitoris, I couldn't wait to make it happen for me. I'll be honest, the first few attempts, it didn't. Then it didn't happen some more. Then something not good began to happen. I began to become frustrated. Why wasn't it happening? Was I wrong? Were my conclusions erroneous somehow? Was I not doing it right? The seed that sprouted as frustration, I will again confess, grew into obsession.

When my partner and I went into the bedroom, the fun that we'd had, all the giggling, tickling, passion and excitement was gone. Instead, I had replaced it with something akin to an obsessive monomania to orgasm during sex. I was Captain Ahab and that orgasm was my white whale. The more it didn't happen, the more I became obsessed with it, the less fun we had, the less relaxed we were and the less likely it was to happen. Looking back, I know now that it was a viscous, self defeating cycle.

I had orgasm tunnel vision and I had it bad. I couldn't see the forest for the trees.

What had happened was that I had lost perspective and in the process, ironically, I had made my goal unobtainable.

My partner and I worked it out and we rediscovered the path we had lost. We got where we wanted to go but we had to have a talk and make a conscious effort to bring back that spark of fun.

There is a lesson in here for any couple trying to apply what I have taught them in this book. Keep your perspective.

I'm going to spell it out for you.

Sex is not about cumming necessarily. Yes, it's a really, really cool part of it. For me. For you. For everyone. But that's not why we should be making love. We should be making love to connect with another person, to laugh, to giggle, to mingle our souls, to feel closeness, warmth, love, touch and desire. We can, honestly, do all of that without orgasm.

My maniacal desire for orgasms during sex had ruined all of that. It'd taken fun and turned into a mundane chore for my lover and I. After that, frustration crept in, grew into obsession and that's not an environment when orgasms, especially the ones this book suggests are possible, happen. They happen when lovers are close, connected, relaxed, aroused and united.

If you choose to play with what I have taught you and see if you can make it happen in your own sex life, my first and most important suggestion to you is to take off your blinders. Keep 'em off and remember that you're there to spend intimate time with and to enjoy the physical comfort of your lover first and foremost.

Pubic Hair Is A Big Help

I'm sure just reading the title of this little section, that you scoffed at me like all my friends did. Yes, I know how popular the Brazilian wax is. Yes, I know how popular it is with the fellas to go bald down there. Sometimes, I'm not sure men know that women naturally have pubic hair or what to do with it if they find it. Yes, bald pussies are so popular that pubic lice have been put on the endangered species list. That's not a joke. Look it up on the internet.

The current state of affairs in women's pubic hair has not always been the case.

As much as it may complicate your efforts to wear a bikini, having pubic hair will help in your efforts to orgasm during sex. Here's why.

Pubic hair serves a purpose. It's not just there like some decorative rug on hardwood floors that should be left bare. It actually serves as a physical means to reduce friction during sex. Here's an exercise to help you get what I'm talking about. Put your hand on the hair on your head. Now, press down with a bit of force and then swirl your hand around. How does it feel?

Other than the pressure, it should feel fine. The hairs literally roll over each other as you do this and keep heat and friction from building up. Now, if you were bald, you would have a very different experience. Your hand would stick and pull the skin and build up heat as you moved it around. Friction would increase. You'd probably get a heat rash if you did it long enough and maybe even some painful chaffing.

Well, that's exactly what happens when you choose to go

bald in the bikini zone and wax all your hair off. The skin loses is natural protection and the sensitive skin in your nethers will get much more heat, friction, chaffing, and heat rash. This is an even bigger problem if you choose to have long bouts of intercourse using the positions I described at the end of the last chapter. Longer sex and less hair can add up to irritation that sends you running to the aloe vera instead of cumming

You can take my advice or you can ignore it. You can't say I didn't mention it. You'll be able to have sex longer, more comfortably and you will have a better chance of orgasming during that sex if you start rocking two hairdos instead of one.

Give This Time

I want you to think back to the second Seeing Is Believing exercise that I gave you. In this exercise, you and your lover worked together to give him an orgasm by stimulating only the corpus cavernosum and corpus spongiosum in the shaft of his penis. If you followed my instructions, you should have ignored the head of his penis altogether.

How long did all of that take relative to say a normal handjob/blowjob that incorporated the glans of the penis?

My guess is that it took a lot longer. Now there was a benefit to this. His mental and physical arousal were probably higher and the resulting orgasm was stronger and more pleasurable. But it <u>DID</u> take longer to get there.

There's another lesson in there for any couple attempting to apply what they've learned in this book to add intercourse orgasms to their sexual routine. That is – give it time.

Just like in that exercise, you (as a couple) will be ignoring the glans of her clitoris and instead will be focusing on the erectile tissues of her internal clitoris. These are sensitive parts, and are, I believe, capable of producing an orgasm, but they are less sensitive than the glans of the clitoris for sure. This will take longer than a normal bout of cunnilingus or a session with a vibrator. Give it time.

Give it time to happen. Show patience. It's a virtue here as much as anywhere else in life. Figure out what positions and movements best stimulate the internal parts of your clitoris and then keep doing them. Slow, steady and consistent stimulation is the key to my orgasms in these situations and I am relatively confident it'll be the key to yours as well. If it feels good, keep doing it. Close your eyes and just keep doing it. Kiss your partner and keep the movements slow, steady and consistent.

The patient, slow, steady, plodding turtle wins this race too.

This Isn't Going To Happen. How 'Bout You Just Eat My Pussy?

There's more than one way for a woman to cum. Don't forget that. That was something that I forgot along the way when my partner and I first started trying to make intercourse orgasms into reality. We would be working together, in a sweaty knot of human flesh, grunting and writhing, and it wasn't happening. Neither of us would say anything. We would both just keep trying even though the ribbon of thought that it wasn't going to happen was in both of our minds. That's how it was in the beginning at least.

Finally, along the way, we both seemed to remember that there were other options. Finally, out of frustration one day, I just suggested a nice round of oral sex instead. He was more than happy to oblige. It was a huge relief to both of us actually. It took the pressure off. We both needed that badly and the resulting orgasm was more than enough to make me smile from ear to ear.

There's a lesson in here too. Failure is going to be part of this experience for you. Most things don't work, or at least don't work well the first time we try them. The first time you rode a bike, I'm sure you fell. I failed my driving test the first time. It wasn't the first Apollo mission that landed a man on the moon. It was the 11th. Long story short, most likely, you aren't going to be successful immediately. You need to be prepared for that and you need to know what to do when that comes up.

It's easy actually. Just suggest that your partner get down and get to work. Just take the pressure off.

If, one the other hand, it's one of those times that your too overstimulated, you feel like you shot past your orgasms and your legs are twitching like a frog in a high school science experiment, be honest, tell him and accept failure with grace. Try again in a few hours or tomorrow. Let your nerves calm down. Failure is a big, ever present part of life and there is nothing wrong with it. At times, we just have to accept it.

The only time you truly fail is when you choose not to try again.

You got back on that bike. I passed my driver's test the third time and man made it to the moon.

The "Gung Ho" Couple

I've always really liked this phrase. Most people associate the phrase "Gung Ho" with something in the military. That's not where it comes from or what it means. It's actually Chinese. I don't know exactly which dialect, but it's Chinese. It means, to translate the idea, "working together". That's it. It simply expresses the idea of working together, as a group, towards a common purpose.

I could not think of a better phrase when trying to apply what you've learned in this book.

You both need to understand that you need to work together as a couple to make this all happen. That means teamwork and teamwork breaks down into communication and trust. Let's take a quick moment to highlight a few thoughts concerning communication and trust.

First, if you, as a couple, really want to do this, you need to agree to talk about it ahead of time. Make that agreement right now, before you ever venture into the bedroom. If you don't, it's going to make things a lot harder, if not impossible. Ladies, he's at a total disadvantage. He has no idea what feels good and what he's supposed to do. You're going to need to explain it to him.

This really means two things. First, when you're experimenting with your internal clitoris and learning how to stimulate it, you're going to need to tell him what you need him to do. This is not a time to be shy. You need to be short. You're going to need to be direct and assertive. You're going to need to put exclamation points on your sentences! Emphasis! You may need to bark orders like a drill sergeant. Trust me here, if he's into what you two are doing (and he will be) this will be a huge turn on to him anyway. I don't mean subtle. I mean barking order like the confident empowered woman you are. Working together does not mean that someone isn't in charge. Someone is always in charge. Ladies you're in charge here and you need to be comfortable owning it.

Men, you need to be good soldiers here and listen to what your sergeant is telling at you. Following orders makes for good teamwork.

Beyond just yelling commands at him, ladies, you should have wrap sessions afterward to let him know how things went. Again, he doesn't know and he needs you to fill him in and answer all the questions swirling in his head. How did it feel? Did you get close? Did you cum? He desperately wants to know these things and much more. Talk about it openly, honestly and directly. Tell him what worked. Tell him what didn't, like if he kept moving. Focus on the positive, but address the negative and improve your performance together. Think of yourselves as a pair of competitive ice dancers working on a routine. They sit down, talk about how things went, criticize each other and work to improve. They never pull of those big finishes the first time. You probably won't be either. There's lots of working towards it and open communication along the way. The same holds true when trying to have orgasms during sex.

Trust is the other big part of teamwork.

When working towards intercourse orgasms, you need to know that you can count on the other person. Ice dancers work as much on trust as they do on their moves. This is a two way street. Men, you need to trust what she's saying and doing. She wants this. She wants this to happen and she's really looking forward to it. Trust her actions, lay back and let her direct the action. Trust her judgment and instructions. Men, I know, are used to being active participants and I am tasking you to perform a very passive role. I know it won't be easy, but you need to let go and trust that she knows what she's doing. Pretend you're on an airplane. When you get on an airplane, you don't know the pilot, you know nothing about them, you know nothing of the plane's mechanics. But you get on there and let all these strangers send you hurtling into space at 500 mph. Usually, you just sit back, trust them and quietly sip your complimentary beverage while thumbing a magazine. Maybe you take a nap. You're trusting them. Do the same thing here.

Ladies, you need to trust your men. They're good guys. They're clearly, very fond of you. Nothing would please them more than for you to be able to cum while having sex with them. Trust them to lie still. Trust them to take direction well and work with you as a team. Trust them enough to give this a try.

I know you might be a little nervous, you might even feel a little bit on display, but trust them to be patient, loving, take direction well and a good team member. If you do, you might be able to walk through a sexual door you never thought you could open. You just have to trust your partner first. It might be a leap of faith, but in the end, I think you'll say that it was worth it.

That's the end of my little spiel about teamwork and the Gung Ho couple. Just keep the spirit of working together in your hearts and heads, and you may be able to go farther than you thought – together.

Foreplay, Foreplay, Foreplay

A woman complaining about foreplay is so cliché, it's barely worth mentioning. However, there are often truths in cliches. The truth is that most couples in this world don't spend enough time focusing on foreplay. I get it. We all lead busy complicated lives and it's so often a fight just to find a few extra minutes in the day. However, foreplay is one of those things, especially in the context of this book, that we just have to make time for.

Few things will help you, as a couple to achieve orgasm during sex, more than foreplay. If you have read this far, you now know a lot more about the clitoris and my conjectures on its role in a woman's orgasm during sex. You also appreciate how it swells and enlarges during sex like a man's penis and you understand, just like a man, a woman needs to be very physically aroused to be able to achieve orgasm. Half aroused is not good enough and you need to do a lot more than just break the plane. You as a couple should plan on going the extra mile.

My partner and I have always put a high emphasis on foreplay, but just like all of you, we're busy. We don't get to spend as much time together as we would like. When we do find ourselves locked in a bedroom together, buttons fly, passions flare and, I will confess, sometimes, foreplay for both of us gets left off the menu. We just can't wait to get to the actual sex.

But I will say, long drawn out, passionate foreplay makes it so much more likely and so much easier for me to cum. The longer the foreplay, the more connected I feel to my lover and the more aroused I am. The sex, the stimulation, the pleasure all feel better, deeper and stronger when we've spent a lot of time rolling around kissing like high schoolers slowly undressing each other. The orgasms are stronger and better too.

I won't go on forever, but I will say and I will advise you to make time for foreplay, especially before you try any of the exercises in this book. Spend a lot of time rolling around, kissing, undressing, laughing, giggling, having fun and the orgasms will most likely come much more often and much easier. They will probably be better when the come too.

Enough said.

A Lot Of This Is Mental

For me, personally, I think a lot of the challenges I faced when working all of this into my love life were mental. I wasn't relaxed enough, I don't know that I was 100%

convinced that I was on the right track. My body had become conditioned to orgasming a certain way, under certain conditions that were different from what I was trying to do. Long story short, there were some mental hurdles that I needed to jump over.

Something that was very helpful for me in getting over all of these mental blocks was bringing a vibrator to bed with me. I went out and bought a very small but very delightful bullet vibrator and I worked it into sex. I would use it while I was on top and the powerful vibrations on the glans of my clitoris would bring about powerful orgasms very quickly with my lover inside of me. This was very helpful for three reasons.

The first was, like most women out there, I wasn't used to having an orgasm during sex. It was always oral sex with my lover in a submissive position, not eye to eye. That wasn't the case with me in the cowgirl position. They were looking right up at me and their eyes were distracting. The first time I came on top of him was hard, but the vibrator offered the sensations that I needed to put me over the top. The next time was easier. After a little while, all of that silly bashfulness (I know how silly and uptight it sounds) and I was used to his eyes on me. Shortly after that, I began to take pleasure in his eyes on me when I was cumming. I'd turned it into something I liked, something I craved, from something that I had been uncomfortable with.

Second, the vibrator also really helped with clit stimulation. With a vibrator right on the glans of my clitoris, the rest of my clitoris was highly, highly stimulated. Men can get half boners, why can't women? The vibrator made sure that I was fully, 100% aroused. In doing so, while playing with the vibrator, I could feel all of the sensations of my clitoris, after a bit of self observation, I had learned what I liked, how I liked it, how to position my body to get the most stimulation possible. Being on top felt better and better until I was able to bring myself to orgasm without the aid of the vibrator.

Conditioning was the last reason that I think the vibrator helped me. We all fall into ruts in life. We find something we like and we stick with it. I think, personally, I had gotten so used to orgasming in ways other than intercourse, that I needed to get used to idea before I could do it without the vibrator. I needed to train my mind to expect orgasms during intercourse. The vibrator became my orgasm training wheels that helped me ride until I had gotten used to being up there. Once that was the case, I could set aside the vibrator and I found I was able to ride and orgasm without it.

Whether or not you choose to bring a vibrator into your bedroom is up to you, but I will say, it was amazingly helpful to me and it might be to you. For the small price we pay for tiny vibrators today, it was well worth it. I recommend a tiny bullet style, ask the woman at the counter, she'll be happy to help you find one that will work for you.

Save The Encouragement

I debated a lot about whether or not to include this little section in this book, but in the end, I decided that it was worth it. It shows, that I'm human, my lover is human and that we did indeed stumble on this path together, before we found success. In the end, the lesson seemed much more important than exposing our flaws.

We were making love, I was on top and we were beginning to explore orgasms during sex and internal clitoral stimulation together. I was excited. He was excited. There had been lots of foreplay. We were both hot and heavy and eager. Lots of heavy breathing. We were having a great time and I was feeling things I had never felt before and I could feel what I hoped would be my first orgasm during sex beginning to blossom. I started making noise as I kissed him.

Then – he did it. He whispered in my ear.

"Cum for me baby..."

Honestly, I think I cringed. It was a cliché line from a porno movie, but more than that, it dumped a load of pressure to perform on my shoulders. The start of the orgasm I'd been feeling disintegrated.

We got into a little bit of a spat at that point. I was mad. I thought this was going to be the day. I was into it. It felt great and I was getting closer than I had before. Then, like an idiot, he "encouraged" me and ruined it all. We argued a little. He apologized. He seemed confused. In the end I did forgive him. But we talked about it.

His intentions, like so many, were good. But the end result was bad. He wanted to encourage me. He likes when I tell him to cum in me and when I encourage him. He didn't get the pressure aspect. I'd put a lot of pressure on myself already. I really wanted it. I didn't need his encouragement, I explained calmly at this point. I felt like he was egging me on to perform and that just soured the whole experience. I told him, what I needed from him was patience and quiet support. We made up. I told him if he needed to do something with his mouth he could smile or kiss me, but, in all honesty, if he felt like saying something he saw in a porno, he should just stay silent.

The lesson in here, I'm including for the guys. Guys, we love you. We really do. We know you want this. We want it too. We want it more than you do. We want the option to come in our lover's embrace like you can. We want to tap into our physical sexuality and experience heightened levels of release at the same time we're one with our partner. We want you to be there when it happens. But what we need from you is quiet, patient love and support. Save the encouraging and pressuring words for some other time.

Like I told my guy, and like I've mentioned before, if you need to do something with your mouth while she's using you like a sexual jungle gym to explore her internal clitoris, smile or kiss her. But keep it to those two things.

Kissing Shouldn't Stop – Ever

Kissing is great foreplay, but it shouldn't stop as soon as he gets the tip wet. That's a huge, common mistake. Kissing should be a constant, ever present part of your lovemaking in general, especially if you, as a couple, are trying to bring about her orgasm during sex. You can never kiss too much.

Let's face it. Kissing pours gasoline on the fires of passion.
I think that's a little bit of a tortured metaphor, but you get
the point. When you're hot and horny and into sex, kissing
only makes it better. You close your eyes, get lost in the
passion and the wonderful, sexy mystery that is kissing and
you get lost somewhere else together. You get out of your
head, turn off the rational part of your mind and exist in a
private world made for two. There's a reasons that poets
have written about kissing since humans learned to write.
Kissing is really cool.

Basically, just keep the kissing going. It'll help quiet your
minds and let you just be in the moment together. Kissing
is amazingly arousing and helps to stimulate our brains as
much as out bodies. When our brains are aroused, it's
much easier to cum as a rule for both genders. Beyond
that, if you're kissing, there's no talking. There's no
misplaced encouragement, rushing or asking if something is
wrong. Also, when we kiss, eyes are usually closed and fears
of being on display are diminished if not eliminated.

Long story short, while you're exploring and experimenting
with what you've learned in this book, you should be kissing
a lot.

Well, There Ya' Have It

In speech classes that I've taken, I always struggled a bit in the closings and it's no different now. I tried to think up something clever to say or some great words to finish on, but I came up short. Instead, I figured I'd just keep it short and sweet.

Throughout this work, I feel that I have been very honest, open and frank. I never claimed to have a monopoly on wisdom, insight or truth. I never stated that any of what I presented was fact. I was clear that this book is one of both conjecture and opinion. However, that being said, I stand by my work. I believe what I wrote. I believe that the basic tenets of the ideas that I set forth are true and correct and much more accurately explain my world observations than the G-Spot ever could.

More than anything, in this book, I wanted to spark debate, thought and the opportunity for women, and men, to consider another option. I wanted to get people thinking in ways that they might not have considered before. I wanted to make you go "huh, I didn't know that" or "wow, that makes a little more sense". I hope, with all my heart that I have done that. I hope with all my heart that you've found this book helpful, thought provoking and useful. I hope, very much, that the information will be useful to you and your partners in creating a richer, deeper, more intimate sex life.

Thank you so much for reading!

-T.K. Hereford